G000140286

THE ESSENCE OF
Aromatherapy

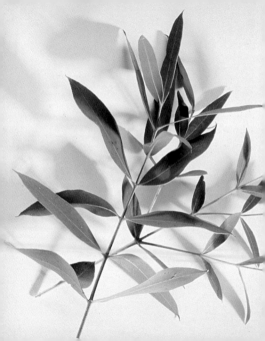

THE ESSENCE OF

Aromatherapy

Paul Lipari

Ariel Books

**Andrews McMeel
Publishing**

Kansas City

www.andrewsmcmeel.com

ISBN: 0-8362-5226-8
Library of Congress Catalog Card Number:
97-74529

Contents

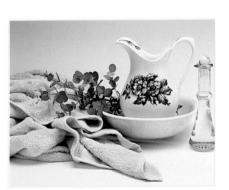

The Essence of Aromatherapy

Aromatherapy was practiced by the Indian, Chinese, and Egyptian cultures of four and five thousand years ago, and its distinguished history continues to this day. It is related to or allied with other venerable medical practices, such as acupuncture, hydrotherapy, and homeopathy, all of which share certain vital principles. The chief of these principles is the idea that when the body (which includes the mind) is in proper condition, everything is in harmony. When that harmony, or balance, is disturbed, illness or injury intervenes. Treatment is then needed to restore nature's balance.

Aromatherapy is exactly what the word suggests: the use of *aromas*, or rather aromatic essences,

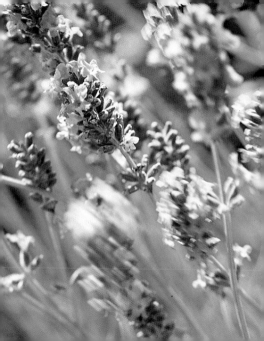

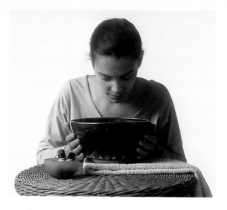

as *therapy*, a way of healing, curing, and toning the body and mind. Aromatic essences are the heart and soul of herbs and plants that give them their smell, their taste, their potency, and any medicinal properties they might contain. They make curry hot; they make coffee beans bitter. They give to camphor those tingling and cool-

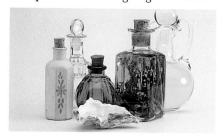

ing qualities that make you feel slightly icy when you have a cold and that instantly clear out clogged sinuses. Rubbing prepa-

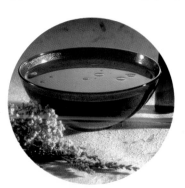

rations of camphor oil on the chest of a cold sufferer is a classic example of aromatherapy—using the essences of aromatic (good- or powerful-smelling) plants to help restore the body's balance. It's no more complicated or arcane than that.

Many of the tenets of aroma-therapy are commonsensical and profound in their simplicity: If a body feels cold, it should be heated, so oil of clove, pimento, or

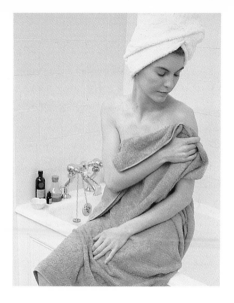

black pepper might be used. If a body feels hot, it should be cooled; camphor or eucalyptus may do the trick. Mint may soothe the stomach; benzoin may soothe the skin. Frankincense can be used to clear mucous membranes, melissa to tone the entire system.

You can bathe in waters steeped in aromatic essences. You can have elaborate body massages in which aromatic oils are rubbed into every pore. You can apply poul-

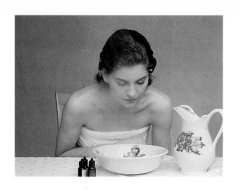

tices marinated in aromatic preparations, inhale vapors compounded of aromatic curatives, burn incense, rub on ointments, get facials with special creams; take baths in special muds, be "fumigated" or "smoked" (similar to sweating in a sauna spiced with aromatic herbs), or drink chamomile tea.

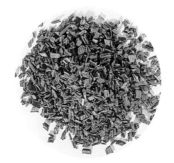

All these, performed properly and with the correct ingredients, are aromatherapy. Burning a cone of incense you bought for ninety-nine cents at the local drugstore may not lead to much, but burning incense prepared with the genuine essence of sandalwood or myrrh could directly affect your psyche, which in turn will affect your body. That is a form of aromatherapy. (And, indeed, even the cheapest incense may make you feel better, more content and more relaxed, merely because it smells pleasant. That is an aroma-therapeutic principle.) Other forms, however, are more classic.

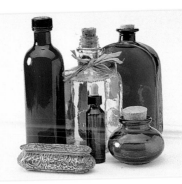

The Mysteries of Scent

Incense has been an integral part of religious ceremonies for many centuries all across the globe, largely because of the soothing effect its smell has on the mind—and the soul.

Temples in India have been historically constructed of sandalwood

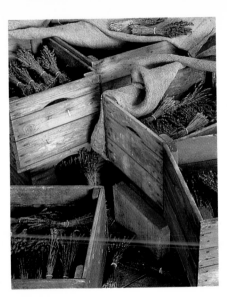

(used to create a celebrated incense throughout the world) not only because of its superior material qualities but also because of the spiritual ones of its scent.

Nubians, who rarely bathe in water because it is so scarce in northern Africa, rub themselves all over with dough and then oil their bodies thoroughly with aromatics. Skin disease is virtually unknown among them, and they're hardly bothered by the cold, cutting winds that sweep through the desert in winter.

In the fourteenth century, the Black Death wiped out half the population of Europe, yet those who dealt in aromatic oils and essences, especially perfumers, were almost entirely unaffected by the plague. Five hundred years later, perfumers again remained immune to the ghastly cholera epidemics raging throughout the world.

To reduce stress and improve

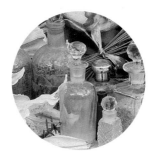

efficiency, Japanese construction firms pipe aromatic essences to their employees through their air-conditioning systems.

Perfumes were banned for a time in eighteenth-century England because they were deemed "too seductive." Women who wore them could even have been prosecuted for sorcery.

Cleopatra is renowned throughout the world as one of history's great temptresses. Some historians believe, however, that she lured men not through any particular physical beauty but through the seductions of her scent. The Egyptian ruler raised the use of perfumes and skin treatment to an art form and owned a vast herbal garden that would be worth millions today. This may have been the true secret of the legendary Queen of the Nile.

What do all these unrelated curiosities have in common? Scents, oils, and aromatic essences. Philosophers, scientists, and medical practitioners have known for thousands of years that various plants and herbs possess mysterious

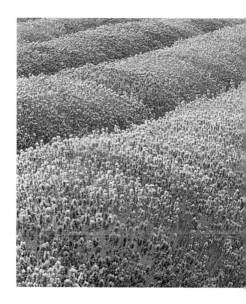

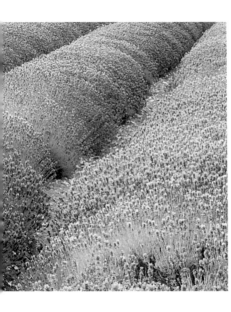

properties, from the tranquilizing to the hallucinogenic, from the poisonous to the sweet. These properties have been tested, explored, examined, philosophized about, and even synthesized throughout the ages, and they've been used in cooking, cleaning, healing, performing religious ceremonies, preparing cosmetics and perfumes, preserving food, and even preserving bodies through mummification.

Why did citizens burn pine branches in the streets of medieval Europe? Because the smoke helped fend off the bubonic plague. What would a Renaissance physician have prescribed to calm your blood (to-

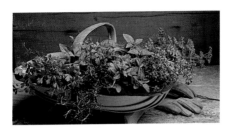

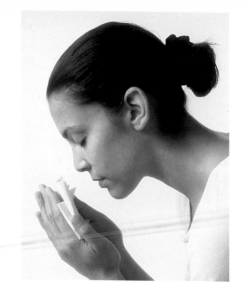

day we'd call it lowering the blood pressure)? Oil of hyssop. Scent is one of the most mysterious of entities, and some scientists and philosophers even believe that the sense of smell may be closely related to the proverbial "sixth sense." It certainly works more quickly on the brain than sight, sound, taste, or touch. When the mystery of scent is harnessed for healing, curing, and restoring the mind and body to fullest efficiency, the process is called aromatherapy. It has been around for thousands of years.

Note: Though aromatherapy may offer relief to many sufferers of aches, discomfort, or general malaise, it cannot necessarily take the place of other treatments. Serious or chronic symptoms and ailments should always be examined and diagnosed by your regular doctor. In addition, only an aromatherapy expert should advise on the proper use of essences; a few essential oils are potentially hazardous under certain conditions.

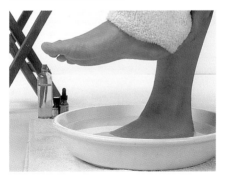

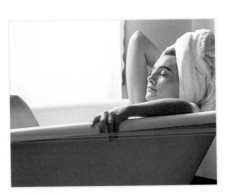

Types of
Therapy

BATHS

You're feeling fatigued. You're feeling depressed. You're nervous and jittery. You're having insomnia and would like to relax (truly relax, relax deep in your body) and get a good night's sleep. Or your joints

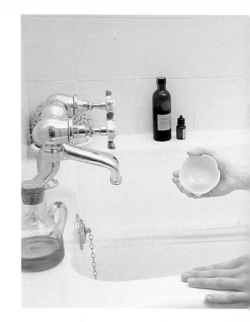

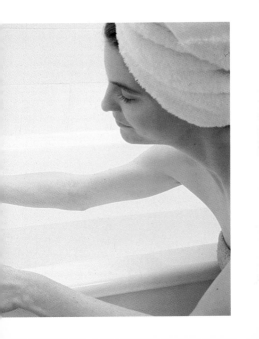

ache, your muscles feel knotted, and your head feels unduly fogged.

You might consult an aromatherapist; at the very least you should study a detailed aromatherapy manual. However, you purchase (or, if you're an expert, you even concoct) an aromatic oil and sprinkle only a few drops in your bath. Then you soak. The aromatic essence, which is so powerful it actually needs dilution in gallons of water so that the body will not be overpowered, permeates you. It cleans your skin, clears your pores, and penetrates your interior.

Your skin, remember, is an organic substance itself. It lives and breathes and allows an oil (though not water) to enter. When that oil courses throughout your body, it slowly, subtly, renders its magic, according to its properties. It may heat you up; it may cool you down. It may awake and arouse you; it may make you sleepy. It may relax your tired muscles, soothe your stomach, or allow you to concentrate or drowse. It can do almost anything, depending on the essence. There's no part of the body it cannot affect, because there's no part of the body it cannot reach.

MASSAGE

After you've taken a bath (an ordinary bath) to cleanse your skin and

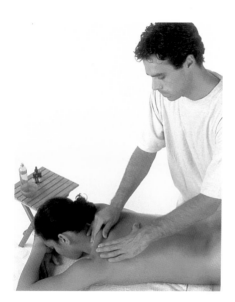

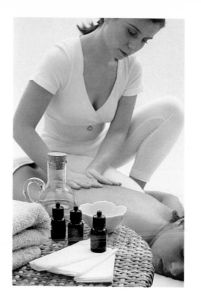

open your pores, you can get a massage, whether elaborate or simple, whether it covers the entire body or concentrates on your tense shoulders or aching calves. As you're massaged, aromatic oils are rubbed into your skin; and, exactly like their counterparts in the bath, they become an invading cavalry to bring you much-needed relief.

Massage is the heart and soul of aromatherapy. Although there are numerous types, all involve the rubbing in of oils. Each brings simple physical pleasure, makes your flesh look and feel better, and smells pleasant; but each also goes deeper, soothing your body and spirit and restoring the balance you need.

SAUNA

You're sweating in a sauna and feel as if all your fatigue, all your blahs, all your "evil spirits" are slowly seeping out of your pores. An ordinary sauna is invigorating, yet an aromatherapy sauna can go further: After you've cooled off, with your

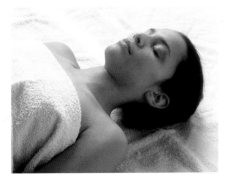

skin in a state of extraordinary receptivity, you'll be oiled and massaged. Your body has "exhaled" unwanted vapors; now it will "inhale" aromatic essences. These penetrate exactly as those of the bath and the massage do. Indeed, they may work even more powerfully.

INCENSE

Incense has been burned at least since Egyptian times, not merely

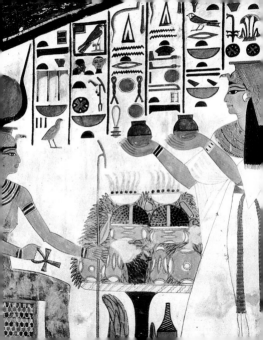

because it smells pleasant, bracing, or hypnotic, but also because it can be both therapeutic and antiseptic. Plutarch, the great biographer of the ancient world, noted that it "lulled one to sleep, allayed anxieties, and brightened dreams"; and an incense recipe from the Ebers papyrus of the Eighteenth dynasty, approximately thirty-five hundred years old, bears a remarkable resemblance to the formula for a modern-day facial pack (still an-

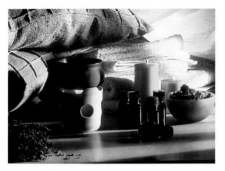

other type of aromatherapy). The high priests of ancient Egypt were history's first true aromatherapists.

Hundreds of recipes abound, each aimed at a different result and state of mind, but in order to effect

real changes in the consciousness
or the body, the incense must be
natural and organic, not compounded of synthetic materials.
Herbalists and aromatherapists
possess almost as many methods as
they do essences, yet the principle
behind them is always the same:
The life force extracted naturally
from selected plants is naturally
introduced into the body, where
it—naturally—does the work of
soothing, relaxing, healing, ton-

ing, and restoring the harmony that was lost. Balance lies at the very heart of it, but nothing will happen if the ingredients are fake.

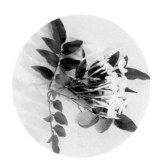

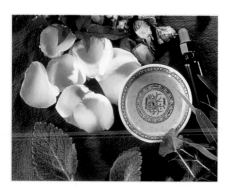

Essential
Questions

❦

1. Where do essences come from?
Essences come from plants—for the
most part the same plants that have
been used throughout the centuries for medicinal and culinary
purposes: geranium plants, clove
trees, juniper bushes, and gal-
banum shrubs, to name a few. The

exact location within each plant depends on the essence. Oil of lavender results from flowers, oil of cinnamon from barks, oil of cypress from cones, and oil of citronella from grass. Fennel oil comes from seeds, eucalyptus from leaves, bergamot from rinds, and calamus from roots. Petals (oil of neroli), twigs (birch), dried flowers (chamomile), pods (garlic), flowering tops (peppermint)—virtually any part of the plant can supply the

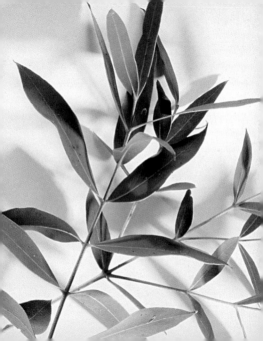

essence. Sometimes the same essence can be extracted from more than one part.

2. How are essences extracted?

The usual method is distillation, in which the plant or plant part is steamed in a vat. The distilled essence (now concentrated and therefore very potent) is cooled. Because it's usually lighter than water, it is easily skimmed off.

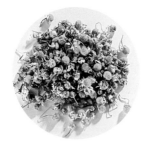

Solvent extraction, often though not exclusively used with flowers, is also common. The flower is soaked in some sort of solvent, usually alcohol, which absorbs the essence. The blend is then distilled, the solvent burns off, and

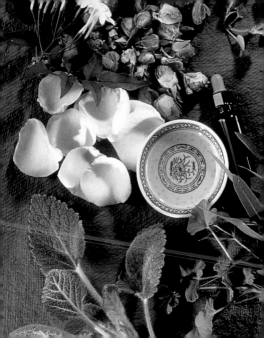

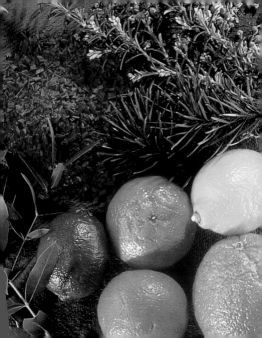

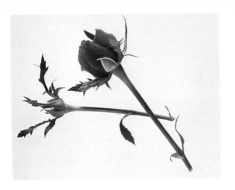

the oil is condensed into what is
called an "absolute."

Other methods exist for certain
plants, but the idea is always the
same: Extract the life essence natu-

rally, and it will retain its potency
for years.

3. What do essences look like?

Many of them look more like water
than oil: They don't have the greasy
characteristics of the oils we are
used to.

Most essences are clear, but a
few, especially the absolutes, are
colored. Lemon oil, as you might
expect, is yellow. Bergamot oil

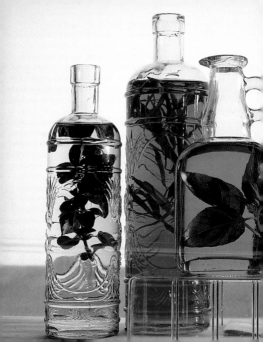

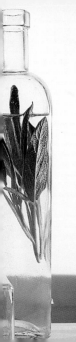

(which imparts to Earl Grey tea its unique and indescribable flavor) is green. Oil of chamomile is blue, and patchouli oil is a rich, reddish brown.

Frankincense and myrrh—heady, heavy, and crucial to the production of incense for thousands of years—are technically

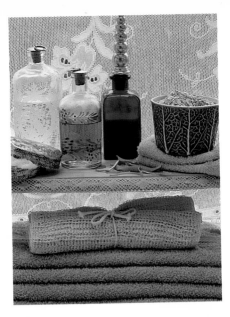

resins, not oils, produced from the gums of their distinctive bushes. Benzoin is also a gum. All are available already dissolved in other mediums. Otherwise they can be purchased in their resinous states and melted down.

4. What do essences smell like?

In most cases, they smell exactly how you would expect them to—rose oil like roses, lavender oil like lavender, and so on—though the scent, in these concentrated states, can sometimes be overwhelming. Some evaporate quickly (eucalyptus oil almost at once); others, like sandalwood, will last almost until the end of time. Patchouli oil actually improves with age, though all oils must be carefully stored in cool, dry places and airtight, dark bottles. Light, heat, air, and moisture can all affect the oil's essence.

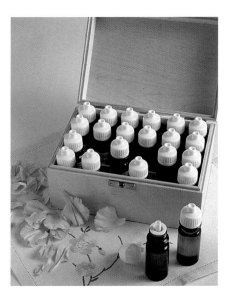

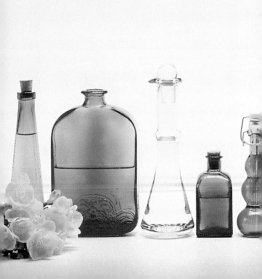

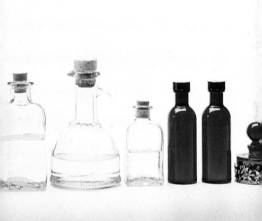

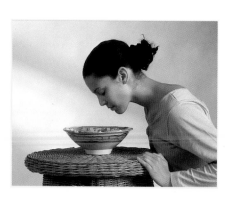

Aromatherapy
Past and Present

Aromatherapy has been practiced
throughout history: from the
Middle East (where the medieval
scientist Avicenna conducted ex-
periments in distillation) to
medieval and Renaissance Europe
(where adventures in aromatics
went hand in hand with attempts

to transform baser metals into gold) to modern Europe and the United States (especially Italy and France, where aromatherapy is widely practiced). It may be more popular now than at any time since the early nineteenth century. And occasionally one cannot help wondering: Is there something these older cultures knew that newer cultures don't?

Even if you can't accept the idea that oil of rose or hyacinth might really sharpen the mind or lily and narcissus put it to sleep, are you not tempted by the idea of an aromatic massage or bath? Wouldn't you rather be surrounded by pleasant natural smells than by chemical aerosols or antiseptics?

If foods contain nutritional essences that can make us healthier and stronger, can't plants contain aromatic essences that might do the same?

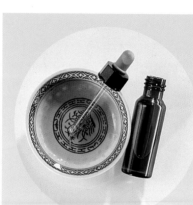

Excellent herbs had our fathers
   of old,
Excellent herbs to ease their
   pain,
Alexanders and Marigold,
Eyebright, Orris, and
   Elecampane.
                    —*Rudyard Kipling*

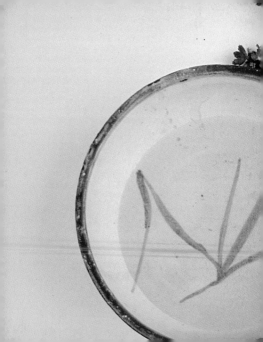

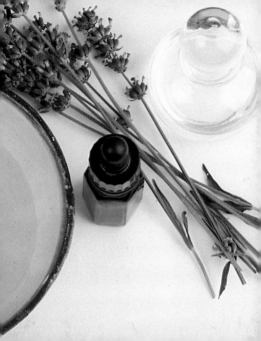

The text of this book is set in
Mrs. Eaves, and designed by
Mspace,
Katonah, New York.

Book design by
Maura Fadden Rosenthal